Wake Up!

A Sensory Stimulation Program for Nursing Home Residents . . .

Pamela Sander, TRS

M & H Publishing Company, Inc.
P. O. Box 268
La Grange, Texas 78945-0268

Printed in the United States of America

First Edition Published 1987

Second Printing 1988
Third Printing 1989
Fourth Printing 1990
Fifth Printing 1991
Sixth Printing 1992
Seventh Printing 1993
Eighth Printing 1994
Ninth Printing 1995

ISBN: 1-877735-14-0

Copyright © 1987 by M & H Publishing Company, Inc. All rights reserved. No part of this publication may be reproduced, stored in a retrieval system or transmitted, in any form or by any means, electronic, mechanical, photocopying, recording or otherwise, without the prior written permission of the publisher.

ABOUT THE AUTHOR

Pamela Sander is a therapeutic recreation specialist registered in Texas with the Texas Recreation and Parks Society and nationally with the National Therapeutic Recreation Society (NTRS), a branch of the National Recreation and Parks Association. Originally from New Orleans, and a graduate of Louisiana State University in Baton Rouge (1968), she was a charter member of the Louisiana Therapeutic Recreation Society and the first Louisiana representative to NTRS's States Advisory Council. Pamela moved to Texas in 1978.

Over the past sixteen years Pamela has traveled the country teaching workshops, seminars and courses on a variety of topics related to working with the elderly, leisure counseling, and activities therapy in long term care, acute care, and residential care facilities. Her work experience includes physical rehabilitation, psycho-social rehabilitation, leisure counseling, as well as long term care social activities programming. Since relocating in Texas, Ms. Sander has taught well over 150 Activity Directors the tools of their profession in the state required 80 hour course for Activity Directors at both College of the Mainland in Texas City (1979) and North Harris County College in Houston (1979 to the present).

Pam, as she prefers to be called by her friends, is currently residing in Houston where she serves as a consultant to approximately eighteen nursing homes and hospitals and is Vice President of Facility Consulting Service, Inc., a private consultant firm for health care facilities. An active member of the Texas Health Care Association's Activity Coordinator's Council, Pam has been instrumental in promoting professionalism and increasing the awareness of the importance of strong activity programs in nursing homes. This is her fourth published text. The first was a joint effort by Mattie Locke, RN, Karen Walton, RD, and Pamela Sander, TRS, entitled Care Plans That Work, 1983, an interdisciplinary preprinted book of "pull" care plans.

Subsequently she wrote the best seller <u>Activity Care Plans for Long Term Care Facilities (or, if you didn't write it down, it wasn't done!)</u> as well as <u>Activity and Volunteer Service Policies and Procedures</u>.

ACKNOWLEDGEMENTS

Many thanks to:

Sandra Dorty, A.D. and Cloteil Bolden, A.D. of American Health Centers, Inc's Hermann Park Manor in Houston, who first asked for my help in developing a program such as this for their 185 residents, many of whom needed some sort of mental stimulation to help them cope with our "reality." Also, for serving as the first test grounds on this progressive program of progression activities for mind-bound residents.

Mr. H. S. and Mrs. A. S. as well as the hundreds of other residents such as these two who have participated and benefitted from this program.

And, finally, to Eddie, who "got behind me and inadvertently stimulated me" to finish this ... merci beaucoups ... cher.

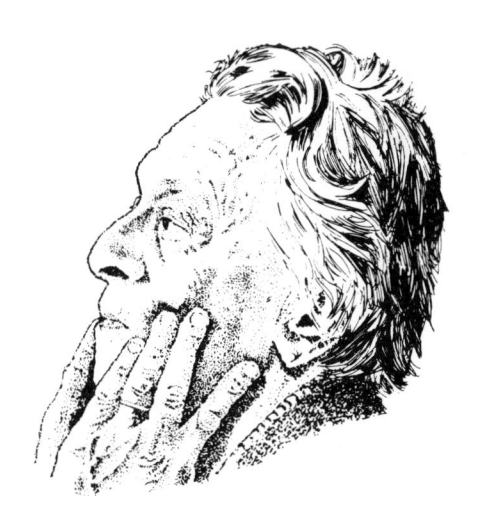

Dear Prudence

Dear Prudence, won't you come out to play.
Dear Prudence, greet the brand new day.
The sun is up, the sky is blue.
It's beautiful and so are you.
Dear Prudence, won't you come out to play?
Dear Prudence open up your eyes.
Dear Prudence see the sunny skies.
The wind is low, the birds will sing
That you are part of everything.
Dear Prudence, won't you open up your eyes?
Look around round
Look around round round
Look around.
Dear Prudence let me see you smile.
Dear Prudence like a little child.
The clouds will be a daisy chain.
So let me see you smile again.
Dear Prudence, won't you let me see you smile?

        the Beatles

TABLE OF CONTENTS

Introduction to the Program	1
A bit of history	1
The plan	2
The wake-up	3
After the "wake-up"	6
Level One	9
Week #1 through Week #6	
Evaluation to proceed	26
Level Two	27
Week #7 through Week #20	
Level Three	47
Week #21 through Week #29	
The Holiday Series	54
Week #30 through Week #37	
People, Members of the Family	60
Week #38 through Week #42	
General Themes	65
Week #43 through Week #52	
Postscript	72
Appendix - Sample forms	75
Weekly Planning Sheet	77
Resident's Participation Record	79

INTRODUCTION TO THE PROGRAM

A bit of history...

In the latter part of May, 1985, I received a phone call from the first of the two ladies working at Hermann Park Manor mentioned in the acknowledgements, Sandra Dorty. At that time Sandra was the chief Activity Coordinator of the 185 bed facility in downtown Houston. Sandra was very upset over comments made during the exit interview by the local Texas Department of Health Social Worker following the re-licensure survey of the nursing home. It seemed the Social Worker, who surveyed the activity and social services programs of the facility, found the activity program to have serious problems regarding meeting the needs of those residents who were suffering from some sort of thought disorder or thought disruption. And, a deficiency was written.

Sandra, an experienced and well qualified Activity Coordinator, recognized that this area of her programming did, in fact, need much attention; but was at a loss as to where to begin. There were nearly eighty-five residents who were classified as falling in that category those of us in health care so conveniently label "confused". Many of these eighty-five residents, nearly half, were semi-bedfast, tube feeders with multiple physical problems. The other ninety or so residents who were active and, for the most part, alert were monopolizing all of her time as well as the majority of the time of Sandra's assistant, Cloteil Bolden.

The Social Worker, in an attempt to be helpful, suggested that Sandra build her volunteer program to handle the alert residents and concentrate her time (Sandra's) and her assistant's time in working with the confused residents. Well, this all sounded good, but remember, this was May of 1985 -- the oil boom that had swelled the pockets of Houstonians in the late

70's and early 80's had already gone bust! Many of the people who once had time on their hands and enjoyed whiling away the hours visiting with nursing home residents during the "boom" years were now out there either looking for paying jobs or already members of the working class. Finding new volunteers to take over the busy program of cooking classes, gardening, discussion groups, exercise, parties, etc., was an extremely difficult task for these two busy Activity Coordinators of this large innercity facility. Those of you reading this who also work in similar settings may be able to identify with this dilemma.

Sandra called me to help her solve this problem. Several years earlier Sandra had been a student in one of my Nursing Home Activity Coordinator classes at North Harris County College. Also during that time, and for the next two years or so, I had served as Sandra's consultant. At the time she called and asked if I could visit to help her with a plan of action to correct this deficiency, it had been almost a year since we had seen each other. I was delighted to once again serve as Activity Consultant to Sandra and looking forward to meeting Cloteil. And, I must admit, intrigued as to how the three of us might be able to plan a program that would work.

After discussing the situation and visiting with a few of these residents, Sandra, Cloteil and I began to map out a program of activities that would include as many of the eighty-five in group situations as possible. We determined that the best approach was to just tackle the situation head-on.

The plan...

Since most of the residents (sixty) needing this specialized program were located on the second floor and were tube-feeders and semi-bedfast, we explored the nursing schedule to determine what times of day would be most feasible to assemble as many residents as possible in a group type setting. The nursing staff, in concern for the skin integrity of these semi-bedfast skilled residents, were in the habit of getting them all up into geri-chairs for a few hours in the morning. Generally, the residents were then wheeled into the hallway to give them a different visual perspective than the four walls of their room. So that by eleven o'clock approximately forty-five to fifty of these residents were up and out of their rooms in the hallways.

As expected, Sandra, Cloteil and I determined that any sort of group programming would best be executed at 11:00 am in the halls. Now that "when" it would occur and "where" it would occur were deter- mined, we were confronted with the "what" that would occur.

We began discussing each of the residents' individual needs, looking for common grounds shared by all. Most were very ill. Most had naso-gastric tubes for feedings (some were hand-fed). Most were semi- alert in that they did seem to be awake, but were not necessarily verbally responsive to others. Most had some sort of disease process working that impaired thinking; many had a stroke or a series of strokes that had caused brain damage, some had Organic Brain Syndrome, some Alzheimer's, some severe head trauma, many had a combination of these in addition to a variety of other diseases that affect the elderly. Many had limited contact with family and/or friends. Most had been retired from their former occupations for several years. Most were in their eighties. All had different interests. All were in need of something pleasant and fun to which they might look forward. All had been unresponsive in varying degrees to individual attempts at gaining their attention and sustaining that attention for any measurable length of time. In other words, all had virtually acquiesced to spending their remaining days in their own world shutting out the attempts of others to penetrate these individual worlds.

The first problem that had to be tackled was to gain the attention of each of these residents. They had to be mentally awakened.

The wake-up...

It was decided that Cloteil, because of her nursing aide experience prior to being promoted to the position of Assistant Activity Director, would be the primary staff person in charge of the new program. When working in the nursing department Cloteil had been assigned to the second floor and had worked with many of these residents. Her knowledge of their physical abilities would come in handy.

The program we mapped out began with a bombardment of the senses. Cloteil was to use as much "sensual noise" as could be mustered. The program would occur every weekday at 11:00 in the hallway where the residents sat. This eliminated any time being wasted gathering residents together in one area. The nursing staff was briefed as to what to expect. Their assistance was requested in placing the residents in the hallway elbow to elbow, chairs touching so that each resident could physically feel the person next to him/her. This is very important, as you will read later on in this chapter.

We decided to begin the program using primary colors. The first week, "blue"; the second, "red"; the third, "yellow". (The actual programs of "what" occurs "when" follow this introduction chapter.) The fourth week, Cloteil moved into the secondary colors. And so the program began.

Cloteil went up to the floor on that first day not really knowing what to expect. She brought with her large sheets of blue poster board and a lot of courage. For 15 minutes, she walked up and down the row of residents shouting, yes shouting, the color's name. "Blue, this is blue. Blue, Mrs. ____, this is blue..." attempting to gain each residents attention. Her efforts were met with extremely limited notice on the part of the residents and much subdued snickering on the part of the staff. Thus she continued until 11:15. She then thanked the residents for their attention and ended the first exercise.

On the second day, Cloteil reminded the nursing staff to place the residents elbow to elbow and began the activity promptly at 11:00. On this day she again used the large sheets of blue paper and added a cassette tape of "Blue Moon." The volume of the music was turned up loud enough that the residents (and anyone else on the second floor) could actually feel the base rhythm. As the music played, Cloteil again went up and down in front of the residents stopping at each one in turn repeating "Blue, this is blue, Mrs. ____... Mr. ____ this is blue, look at the blue... feel the blue in the music..."

On the third day, Cloteil added a blue, silk scarf. As the music played she encouraged each resident to touch the scarf, placing it in their hands and rubbing their faces gently with the scarf.

Thursday's additions included blueberry jam. As the music played, after each resident had an opportunity to feel the scarf and hear Cloteil's description of the "feel" of the scarf and the "feel" of the music, Cloteil then introduced the blueberry jam. She had individual coffee stirs which she dipped into the jam jar encouraging each resident to smell the jam. Then she gently placed just a speck of jam on each resident's lips. This created attention. Carefully Cloteil noticed one or two tongues slowly licking the sweet jam.

Thus the program continued; the "blue" week became a "red" week, then "yellow". After five or six weeks of this very basic program Cloteil began to notice subtle changes in each resident's response. Some began tapping wiery fingers on the lap boards that protected them from falling forward in their geri-chairs. Others began to give eye contact as soon as they heard Cloteil's voice. Still others seemed to actually be paying attention and attempting to answer Cloteil's questions about the color theme for the week. The residents on the second floor were "waking-up". They were becoming mentally alert to the activity going on around them!

Cloteil also began to notice subtle changes in the attitude of the staff on that floor. She saw nursing assistants, who had always talked to the residents, take more time in the talking and waiting for the residents to respond. Some began to do so. After about two months into the program, one resident, Mrs. A. S. began talking after nearly seven years of silence. Her conversations didn't always make sense, but that was not important. What was important was the fact that she was talking and laughing and seemingly taking a greater interest in her surroundings.

Another resident, Mr. H. S., whose attention span only lasted from one cigarette to the next, began following the program. In the beginning he could hardly sit still long enough to finish a cigarette he had started, before asking for his next one.

His entire world centered around smoking. About six months into the program Mr. S. was paying attention and not smoking during this activity. He was answering questions, singing along to the music and even remembering the words to songs that he sang years ago. In the first year of this program his attention span grew from what was probably less than three minutes to more than one hour in an activity.

One of the most interesting effects noted during the initial "wake-up" program was the way in which the residents seemed to be responding to each other. The urge to "compete" with their "elbow neighbors" for Cloteil's attention seemed to serve to speed the responses of some. It was as if the sheer number of residents in each session was a factor in the re- sponses gained. Cloteil and Sandra were pleased. By the time the Department of Health Social Worker returned in ninety days to check on the deficiency, it was a very different scene on second floor. Prior to the program beginning, when you got off the elevator on second floor, it was as if you were on a hospital floor -- the only real noises heard were that of the staff going about their daily routine. After the initial twelve weeks, there were noises on second floor, people noises -- conversations, laughter, music, and of yes, some moaning and crying, but people noises, not hospital noises.

Needless to say the deficiency was cleared.

After the "wake-up"...

Now that the residents were mentally "awake," Cloteil began adding themes to the program that required the residents to think and do some problem solving. The problems, at first, were very simple, for example -- showing a picture of a bicycle, Cloteil would ask "What is this? . . . Yes, that's right . . . Tell me something about a bicycle . . ."

And so the program continues today, each week themes of varying complexity are added. One of the really great aspects about this program is that new people added can enter at the level of the group. With just a little extra attention in the begin-

provements as Mrs. A. S. or Mr. H. S., but they all do accomplish one thing -- they all have fun with it. Wouldn't it be nice to know that when you turn 85 you can have something fun to look forward to every morning!?!

In the pages that follow you will find approximately five months of detailed programming followed by a list of theme ideas that can carry you through the first year. It is recommended that you follow the first five or six weeks programs carefully. After that, move at whatever speed your residents can handle. Have fun with this program. Believe in it. If <u>you</u> enjoy it and <u>you</u> believe in it, it will work -- it will. Nothing is more important to the success of this program than your desire to see it succeed.

LEVEL ONE

Each of the following sets of weekly themes contains the name of the theme, the objective for the week, the materials needed for the week and, in the first 20 weeks or so, detailed instructions of how to proceed with the week.

It is suggested that before beginning the week, you have gathered all the materials you may need to proceed. Each week has suggested "theme" music or sounds. I recommend you use a tape recorder for this music. Many public libraries have tapes available to loan. Other sources for the music may include:

1. your own music library or that of family and/or friends

2. church music libraries

3. high school choirs -- you may solicit their assistance by asking them to sing whatever is necessary while you tape them.

4. your own voice . . . (it is not important that your music be of grammy award quality, only understood and heard by your residents).

The "flashing light" referred to in this first level may be:

1. a portable strobe light with colored gels attached in front;

2. a flash light with colored cellophane attached, that you click on and off manually; or,

3. a color wheel (as is often used to illuminate Christmas trees) for which you have prepared the different colored gels.

Gels may be purchased at theatre supply stores or through catalogs that supply theatres. If you are located in an area where these purchases may be difficult, check with your local high school theatre department. They may be willing to give or loan you the equipment needed.

WEEK # 1

THEME: Blue

OBJECTIVE: Residents will be able to identify the color blue and objects that are blue or have blue in their names.

MATERIALS TO BE GATHERED:

Vision - blue gels for flashing light, sheets of blue construction paper, lengths of blue fabric

Hearing - (music) "Blue Moon", "Blue Christmas", "Blue Birds", etc.

Touch - blue colored scarfs, blue flowers, box blueberries

Smell - blueberry jam

Taste - blueberry jam (prepared in fluted med cups)

MONDAY'S PLAN:

Wrap self in blue fabric, use either blue flashing light and/or the large sheets of blue paper. Go to each resident in the group and flash light or rattle paper near face - gain eye contact, keep repeating "Blue, blue...", encourage same response from each resident. Reward appropriate response with praise. Ask questions like "Mrs. S., tell me something about the color 'blue'."

TUESDAY'S PLAN:

Repeat the dress and flashing lights of Monday. Add music, be sure the volume is loud enough to be heard as well as felt, i.e., residents who may have a hearing problem should be able to feel the pulse beat (bass) of the music.

WEDNESDAY'S PLAN:

Repeat the dress, flashing lights and music. Add colored scarf or flowers or box of blueberries. Talk about the item with each resident. Allow them to feel the different textures of the items chosen. Talk about the textures. Encourage the resident to also talk about the objects.

THURSDAY'S PLAN:

Repeat the dress, lights, and music. Return with the blue object. Let the resident feel the "blue". Use the blueberries (frozen or fresh), encourage the resident to roll the blueberries in his/her hands. Have medicine cup (small fluted cups) of blueberry jam on hand with enough coffee stirs to have one for each resident. Encourage each resident to smell the jam (or crush one or two berries and encourage each resident to smell the crushed berries). Let each resident have a taste of the jam on the end of a coffee stir. Talk about the taste. Encourage each resident to express how the jam tastes to him/her.

FRIDAY'S PLAN:

Repeat Thursday.

EVALUATION OF THE WEEK:

Record each resident's overall response to the week's program. Ask yourself the following questions about each resident's responses:

1. Was there eye contact; did the resident follow my movements with his eyes?
2. Was the resident able to verbalize? ... the color's name, ... the name of the objects, ...etc.
3. Was the resident moving to the sound (feel) of the music? Was there a rhythm or pattern to this movement?
4. Was there a reaction to the odor of the jam? ... to the taste? If yes, what?
5. Did the resident seem to have enjoyed the week?

WEEK # 2

THEME: Red

OBJECTIVE: Resident will be able to identify "red" and be able to verbalize "red".

MATERIALS TO BE GATHERED:

Vision - red gel for flashing light; length of red fabric; pictures of red apples; red fire engine, red shoes, etc.

Hearing - (music) "Red, Red Robin", "Red River Valley" (if upbeat)

Touch - apple, red ball, red rose, red ribbons, etc.

Smell - sliced apple (applesauce); cinnamon "red hots"; red rose

Taste - applesauce (might wish to spice this with a dash of cinnamon) (pre-prepared in fluted med cup) for Friday -- applesauce in cups and crushed "red hots" in cup.

MONDAY'S PLAN:

Drape self in length of red fabric, use the red gel on the flashing light, bring out each of the red colored objects one at a time. Place the object in each resident's field of vision, clearly repeat the name of each object, encouraging each resident to repeat after you.

TUESDAY'S PLAN:

Repeat flashing light, and red drape -- add music -- choose one of above suggestions or your own; play music loudly. Again bring out the red objects, one at a time, placing each in the resident's field of vision. Repeat the item's name, encourage each resident to repeat after you.

WEDNESDAY'S PLAN:

Repeat Tuesday's plan. Today as each object is brought out, allow each resident time to hold each object. Encourage the resident to repeat the name of the object or the color "red." Use much praise when a resident gives a correct response.

THURSDAY'S PLAN:

Repeat Wednesday's plan. Have some medicine cups (fluted pill cups) on hand with a teaspoon or two of applesauce in them. Have the cinnamon "red hots" on hand. Encourage each resident to smell the two different foods and identify the smells. Using your supply of coffee stirs, let each resident taste the applesauce. Encourage the residents to verbalize "Ripe, red apples make applesauce..."

FRIDAY'S PLAN:

Repeat Thursday. You may wish to add allowing each resident to taste the cinnamon "red hots". (Crush three or four ahead of time using a pill crusher. The taste the residents might have would be a touch of the powdered candy on the end of a coffee stir.) Use discretion in adding this tasting of the "red hots."

EVALUATION OF THE WEEK:

Record each resident's overall response to the week. Ask yourself the following questions about each resident's response:

1. Was there eye contact? Did the resident track my movement with his/her eyes?

2. Was the resident moving to the beat of the music?

3. Did the resident hold the objects given him/her?

4. Was there a response to the taste of the applesauce? ... the "red hots"?

5. Did the resident verbalize the word "red"? If yes, at what point during the week? If not, did he/she seem to try?

6. Did the resident seem to have a pleasant experience this week? How did he/she convey that message?

WEEK # 3

THEME: Yellow

OBJECTIVE: Resident will be able to identify yellow and choose the yellow object from a grouping with two other colors.

MATERIALS TO BE GATHERED:

Vision - yellow gel for flashing light; length of yellow fabric; yellow rose; banana; pictures of yellow bird

Hearing - (music) "Yellow Rose of Texas" (yes, the author is partial to her adopted state)

Touch - banana, rose, yellow ball (may be a ping pong ball painted with yellow enamel paint), stuffed yellow bird (soft), 2 or 3 objects that are red and/or blue (apple, blueberries, etc.)

Smell - banana, yellow rose

Taste - banana (smashed, served in fluted med cup), grated cheddar cheese (for Friday)

MONDAY'S PLAN:

Drape self in yellow fabric; turn on the yellow flashing light; bring out the chosen objects one at a time. Place each in turn in each resident's field of vision, talking about each object using the name of the object and the resident's name frequently. Encourage the resident to repeat the object's name.

TUESDAY'S PLAN:

Repeat the dress and flashing lights. Add the music. You may be partial to your own favorite song that has "yellow" in it's title, example: "Tie a Yellow Ribbon ... ", "Yellow Submarine", etc. As with weeks 1 and 2, be sure the volume is loud enough to be felt as well heard. Again, bring out the yellow objects one at a time using particular emphasis on the object mentioned in the music. Encourage each resident to repeat the name of the object after you or to sing-a-long with the words of the song.

WEDNESDAY'S PLAN:

Repeat as for Tuesday. Add: when the objects are brought out today, let each resident hold the objects in turn. Discuss the feel and texture of the object. Place emphasis on the banana today to prepare for Thursday. Introduce the red and/or blue objects. Discuss the contrast between the yellow objects and the red/blue objects. Encourage each resident to pick up and hold or point to the yellow object.

THURSDAY'S PLAN:

Repeat the preceding three days, i.e., the dress, the flashing light, the music, the objects for discussing and holding. Add: tasting the smashed banana. Use your coffee stirs, one stir for each resident to prevent cross contamination. Discuss the texture of the whole banana in the hand, and the texture of the banana pulp on the tongue; discuss the smell and the taste. Encourage residents to verbalize their thoughts.

FRIDAY'S PLAN:

Repeat Thursday's plan "en toto". Add: a taste of grated cheddar. Compare the taste to the banana. Ask the resident to identify the banana when paired with an apple and a box of blueberries. (Pictures of the banana, the apple, and the blueberries may be used.) Encourage each resident to respond. Reward appropriate responses with much verbal praise. Remember: Always use each resident's full name when encouraging responses. Example: "Mrs. Ida Smith, show me the picture of the banana, point to the yellow banana, Ida Smith."

EVALUATION OF THE WEEK:

Record each resident's overall response to the week. Ask yourself the following questions about each resident's response:

1. Did the resident look up when hearing his/her name? Was there eye contact during his/her special turn? Did the resident track my movement with his/her eyes?

2. Did the resident respond to the music? Did he/she move with the beat? ... attempt to sing-a-long? ... etc.

3. Did the resident hold the object when placed in his/her hands? Did resident attempt to verbalize response to questions regarding texture and shape of the object?

4. Was resident able to identify the smashed banana by smell? ... by taste? Did resident identify the cheese?

5. Was the resident able to identify the banana when grouped with the apple and the blueberries?

6. Did the resident have fun this week? Does he seem to look forward to these morning exercises?

WEEK # 4

THEME: Green

OBJECTIVE: Resident will be able to identify green and choose the green objects from a grouping with two other colored objects.

MATERIALS TO BE GATHERED:

Vision - green gel for flashing light; length of green fabric; objects that are green: green painted ball, green plant, green limes, green grapes, green lettuce, etc.; green nerf ball

Hearing - (music) "Green, Green Grass of Home" "Greensleeves", "Little Green Apples"

Touch - green ball, green grapes, green limes

Smell - cut lime

Taste - lime juice or lime koolade or lime sherbet in fluted med cups

MONDAY'S PLAN:

Wrap self in green fabric; use the flashing light with the green gel. Bring out two or three green objects - one at a time. Gain each resident's attention by using his/her name. Show one object at a time to each resident. Talk about the object. Ask simple questions: "Can we eat grapes?" "Can we eat this plant?" Reward appropriate responses with much praise. Be sure each resident has had an opportunity to speak.

TUESDAY'S PLAN:

Repeat dress, lights, have objects ready. Add music, keep volume up. Talk about each object. Then focus on the lime, passing it back and forth to each resident in time with the music. The slower pace of most of the recommended selections is conducive to rhythmic passing of the lime - tossing a green nerf ball also works well. Encourage each resident to respond by repeating the name of the object or singing along with the music.

WEDNESDAY'S PLAN:

Repeat Tuesday, i.e., dress, lights, music, and objects. When working with the objects today discuss the shapes. Compare the shape of the lime to the shape of the plant leaves. Let each resident feel the different texture of the objects. Encourage each resident to verbalize the "feel" of each object.

THURSDAY'S PLAN:

Repeat the preceding three days. Add smell today with a lime that has had it's peeling scored slightly to release the natural oils that are contained in the skin. Add taste by using the coffee stirs to hold a small amount of lime juice which is then released on each resident's lips and/or tongue. Encourage residents to discuss objects, taste, smell, etc. Pull on resident's memory of preceding week and compare taste of lime to that of banana.

FRIDAY'S PLAN:

Repeat Thursday "en toto". Bring out pictures of apple, banana, and lime. Ask residents to choose the lime. Bring out pictures of a green plant, a colored plant, and a flowered plant (dogwood in bloom, tulip trees in bloom, etc.). Ask each resident to choose the picture of the green plant. Reward appropriate responses with much praise.

EVALUATION OF THE WEEK:

Record each resident's overall response to the week. Answer the following questions on each resident:

1. Was eye contact present today? Did resident look up and seem to pay attention as soon as the exercise began, or did the resident wait to hear his/her name? Was there a general tracking of my movement?

2. What was the response to the music? ... to his/her name? ... to names of objects? Does the resident seem to pay attention to the music? ... attempt to sing-a-long? ... etc.

3. Was the resident willing to hold the lime? ... pass it back and forth? ... feel the texture and compare it to the texture of the other objects used?

4. Did the resident verbalize at all? Was he able to choose the correct objects when quizzed? ... point? ... answer with his eyes? ... with his voice?

5. Did the resident have fun today? If yes, how did he convey this message to you? If no, what happened?

WEEK # 5

THEME: Purple

OBJECTIVE: Resident will be able to identify purple and name one object that is colored "purple".

MATERIALS TO BE GATHERED:

Vision - purple gel for flashing light; length of purple fabric; purple objects: dark concord grapes, iris bloom, lilacs, purple ball, violets

Hearing - (music) "Deep Purple", "Flying Purple People Eater", "Purple Haze"

Touch - grapes, ball, lilacs, iris blooms, violets

Smell - violet candies, grapes, grape jelly, lilacs

Taste - grape jelly in fluted med cups; violet candies crushed by pill crusher in fluted med cups

MONDAY'S PLAN:

Drape fabric around self; use the flashing light with the purple gel. Use one or two of the purple objects, one at a time. Gain residents attention with the light. Show the object. Talk about shape, color, etc. Ask simple questions. Example: Are these grapes like the green grapes from last week? Reward appropriate responses with much praise.

TUESDAY'S PLAN:

Repeat Monday's plan. Add music. Begin clapping your hands. Encourage residents to follow your lead. Assist those who have difficulty beginning by holding their hands and clapping with them. Each time the word "purple" occurs in the music, emphasize it by waving one of the purple objects in the air. At the end of the music bring out all the purple objects and talk about each in turn. Encourage residents to talk about the objects by asking questions such as: "Mr. Smith, tell me something about grapes ..."

WEDNESDAY'S PLAN:

Repeat Tuesday's plan, i.e. dress, lights, music, objects. Today let each resident hold the objects. Talk about shape, texture, size, etc. Encourage each resident to verbalize the name of each object held. Next, take two objects, for example the grapes and one of the flowers. Play a game with each of the residents by asking them to point to or pick up one by name. Example: "Mr. Smith, point to the grapes ..."

THURSDAY'S PLAN:

Repeat the preceding day's plan. Add smell today by peeling and/or smashing one of the grapes (or having a small amount of grape jelly or grape juice in a cup), having some of the violet candies in a cup, or having a fresh lilac (or silk lilac with lilac scented spray on it). Add taste by allowing each resident to identify the different smelly things and rewarding with a small taste of the edibles on the end of a coffee stir. Compare taste of grape jelly to violet candies. Play the game again with the objects. Use three different objects today.

FRIDAY'S PLAN:

Repeat Thursday. When at end of session playing the selection game, ask each resident in turn to identify the objects verbally. Reward correct responses with much praise. Remember: Always use the resident's full name when addressing each individually.

EVALUATION OF THE WEEK:

Record each resident's response to the week's program. Answer the following questions:

1. Is the amount of eye contact increasing? Is he/she now looking up throughout the entire activity?

2. Was he/she able to maintain clapping to the music after started by me? Did he/she begin clapping on his/her own?

... attempt to sing-a-long to music?

3. Was the resident able to choose the correct objects successively? ... one out of three times? ... two out of three?

4. Was he/she able to call the name of the objects? ... one? ... two? ... three? ... all?

5. Was there "joy" in this week's activity, i.e., did he/she seem to have fun? ... enjoy his/her moment of individual attention?

WEEK # 6

THEME: Orange

OBJECTIVE: Resident will be able to identify "orange" and name three objects that are colored orange. Resident will be able to move to the next level of stimulation program.

MATERIALS TO BE GATHERED:

Vision - Orange gel for flashing light; length of orange fabric; oranges; pictures of oranges growing on trees; orange shapes, pumpkins, decorative gourds, etc.

Hearing - (music) Florida orange juice song, Halloween songs with word "orange" in them

Touch - oranges, decorative gourds, pumpkins

Smell - orange with skin slit to release oils

Taste - orange juice

MONDAY'S PLAN:

Drape self in orange fabric; turn on flashing light with orange gel; use one or two of the orange objects: one at a time. Gain residents attention with the light. Show the object. Talk about the color, shape, etc. Ask simple questions: "Mr. John Smith, can you tell me the name for this?" Reward appropriate answers with much praise.

TUESDAY'S PLAN:

Repeat Monday - dress, lights, objects. Add: music. Emphasize the word "orange" each time it is mentioned in the song. Begin clapping hands, encourage residents to follow suit. Help those who need help. Work all the way through the music. Play song again, now encourage residents to march (or swing legs) in time to music. Again, help those who need assistance to begin (this is good for circulation). Bring out the objects. Talk about each in turn. Ask simple questions. Encourage each resident to participate by asking each a question at his/her level of proficiency. Always remember: Reward correct responses with much verbal praise.

WEDNESDAY'S PLAN:

Repeat Tuesday. When discussing the objects today, allow residents to hold them, one at a time. Discuss texture as well as colors and shapes. Also, discuss uses for the objects. Example: oranges - eating, drinking (source of Vitamin C), flavoring, etc. Reward appropriate responses with praise.

THURSDAY'S PLAN:

Repeat Wednesday's plan. Add "smell" with the whole orange that has had the skin lightly slit in a few spots to release the oils; and "taste" with prepared orange juice (or sliced and peeled orange sections). Provide each resident with a whiff of the whole orange. Encourage to identify the smell verbally. Then provide each with a taste of the orange juice on the end of their individual coffee stirs. Again, encourage each resident to identify the taste. Bring out all of the orange objects. Ask each to identify the objects. Reward appropriate answers with much praise.

FRIDAY'S PLAN:

Repeat Thursday's plan. During the music be sure to pay particular attention to the word "orange" and the object to which it refers. When performing the "taste" and the "smell" portions, emphasize the whole orange. Then bring out all the objects and ask each resident to identify the objects. Reward appropriate responses with much praise.

EVALUATION OF THE WEEK:

Record each resident's response to the week's program. Answer the following questions:

1. Was he/she able to clap to the beat of the music unassisted? ... able to march in place unassisted?

2. Was he/she able to identify the odor of the orange? ... the taste of the orange juice?

3. Was he/she able to identify, by name, at least one of the orange objects? ... two? ... three? ... four? ... all of them?

4. Did he/she seem anxious for the activity to begin? ... smiling at the start? ... eyes tracking movement?

5. Did he/she seem to enjoy the activity? ...respond when called on to do so? ... smile during individual attention?

EVALUATION TO PROCEED TO THE NEXT LEVEL

At the end of these first six weeks your residents should be ready to move on to the next level. It does not matter if all are not functioning at the same level of response. If the majority of the group (more than half) is responding appropriately 70% of the time or more, it is time to move to Level Two: General Concrete Themes.

If the majority of the group is not responding appropriately at least 70% of the time, go back to "Week 1" and begin again with the same progression. At the end of this second six weeks period proceed to Level Two regardless of the residents' responses. The reasoning behind this recommendation is to prevent you, the Activity Director, from becoming bored with the program. If you become bored, your residents will pick up on this and also become bored. Remember: Have fun with this program. Your residents will enjoy you and have fun, too. And, if they are having fun then half the battle has been won -- you will have their attention.

LEVEL TWO

WEEK # 7

THEME: Shelter - Housing

OBJECTIVE: Resident will be able to name three kinds of housing.

MATERIALS TO BE GATHERED:

Vision - slides/pictures of houses, townhomes, apartment buildings, tents, caves, etc.

Hearing - (music) "This Old House"

Touch - Children's toy houses, piece of wood, brick, pieces of carpet

Smell - piece of carpet, piece of wood (painted recently), pot of herbs boiling nearby on a hot plate. Herbs and spices that work well together: cinnamon sticks, bay leaves, whole cloves.

Taste - ginger cookies shaped like a house (Pepperidge Farm)

MONDAY'S PLAN:

Show slides/pictures. Talk about the different types of shelter in the pictures. Insure each resident is paying attention by using their names frequently. Ask simple questions: "Mr. John Smith, did you live in a house? Tell me about your house?" Reward responses with praise.

TUESDAY'S PLAN:

Repeat Monday's plan through to the questions to each resident about their own homes. Then add the music. Move with the beat of the music, encourage residents to follow your lead. Work arm extension movement into your routine. Assist those residents who may need help starting. End with everyone clapping hands as in "applause for job well done".

WEDNESDAY'S PLAN:

Repeat Tuesday up to the point of beginning the movement to music. Before starting this portion of the day's exercise add the objects gathered for touching - one at a time. Let each resident hold them in turn. Talk about texture, where the objects might be found in a home, etc. Then proceed with the music and movement, etc. Don't forget to end with the "applause for a job well done."

THURSDAY'S PLAN:

Repeat Wednesday. When you've reached the portion of the plan where you have each resident hold the objects encourage them to smell each one in turn. Introduce a pot of steaming herbs after the smelling of the carpet, wood, etc., takes place. Then proceed with the music and movement. Don't forget the "applause" at the end. Then add the added reward of the ginger cookie shaped like a house. Emphasize that while one does not normally eat a house, these little houses were made to be eaten. Be sure to have water on hand to offer residents while eating the cookies. Remember that the mouth of an older person is not able to produce enough saliva to keep it fluid while eating a dry cookie. Be sure to stay with your residents until they have finished their treats to guard against choking.

FRIDAY'S PLAN:

Repeat Thursday "en toto."

EVALUATION OF THE WEEK:

Record each resident's overall response to the week. Answer the following questions about each resident:

1. Did he/she show attention when the slides/ pictures were shown? ... able to identify the different types of houses? ... answer simple questions about his/her own home?

2. Did he/she move easily to the music? ... seem to enjoy being touched during the ROM to the arms? ... applaud upon given instructions to do so?

3. Did he/she recognize the different objects shared? ... verbalize their names? ... etc.

4. Was he/she able to smell the objects? How did he/she make you aware of this? ... verbally? ... with gestures?

5. Did he/she enjoy the cookie? Was he/she able to eat it without assistance? Did he/she seem to have fun this week?

WEEK # 8

THEME: Water

OBJECTIVE: Resident will be able to name three places where water is found.

MATERIALS TO BE GATHERED:

Vision - pictures of rivers, lakes, waterfalls, the ocean, etc. Use large pictures and/or slides.

Hearing - (music) "Old Man River", "Raindrops Keep Falling on my Head", make a tape of water being poured into a container, water rushing out of a faucet, a toilet flushing, rain falling, etc.

Touch - containers of water, one for each resident

Smell - tap water, bottled water - in small cups, one of each for each resident

Taste - tap water, bottled water, slivers of ice

MONDAY'S PLAN:

Show pictures (slides are best because the focal point is easily found). Play tape of water sounds. Talk about the pictures. Play game of naming lakes, rivers, etc., that are local to your area. Encourage residents to play the game with you. Use resident's full name and ask simple questions about the different waterways.

TUESDAY'S PLAN:

Repeat Monday's plan. Add music. Move in place to the beat of the music. Encourage residents to follow the beat of the music. Encourage residents to follow your lead; clap hands, kick legs, stretch arms, etc., whatever the mood of the music fosters. Play the game again about the local waterways. Ask questions; encourage residents to respond. Reward appropriate responses with much praise.

WEDNESDAY'S PLAN:

Repeat Monday and Tuesday. Add during the slide show or picture presentation: small bowls of warm water for each resident to feel while the pictures are discussed. Encourage the residents to submerge their fingers in the warm water. Talk about the feel, the temperature, the color, etc. Follow by removing the bowls and starting the music. Move to the rhythm and mood, then continue as on Tuesday with the movement exercise and then the game of naming different waterways.

THURSDAY'S PLAN:

Repeat Wednesday through the fingers being submerged in water. At this point add the sniff and taste. Give each resident small cup of tap water and bottled water. Encourage each resident to smell the two different cups of water. Talk about each - one from a bottle (might wish to use carbonated water), one from the tap. Then have the residents taste each of the waters. Talk about the difference in taste. Continue with the previous days exercise with the music followed by the game of naming waterways.

FRIDAY'S PLAN:

Repeat Thursday's plan "en toto". When tasting the different cups of water, add a third cup with slivers of cracked ice. Discuss the coldness of the ice and how it melts in the warm environment of the resident's mouth. Ask the resident which he/she prefers - the tap water, the bottled water, or the frozen water (ice). Then continue with the music, movement, and game.

EVALUATION OF THE WEEK:

Record each resident's overall response to the week's plan. Answer the following questions about each resident's response:

1. Did he/she track my movement with his/her eyes? ... seem to pay attention?

2. Did he/she submerge his/her fingers in the water following verbal instruction? ... after being shown? Did he/she leave his/her fingers in the water after I moved away to the next resident? ... or pull them out as soon as the one to one attention ended?

3. Was he/she able to recognize the different types of waterways? ... rivers? ... lakes? ... ponds? ... oceans? ... etc. Was he/she able to name any local waterways?

4. Did he/she notice a difference between the bottled water and the tap water? ... taste? ... smell? Did he/she verbalize this?

5. Did he/she show any signs of enjoyment during this week's exercises? Did he/she move with the music, clap hands, etc.?

6. Did he/she seem to have fun?

WEEK # 9 AND WEEK # 15

THEME: Food

OBJECTIVE: Resident will be able to verbalize his/her favorite food.

MATERIALS TO BE GATHERED:

Vision - pictures/slides of people eating foods - many different slides; also pictures/slides of different kinds of food

Hearing - (music) "Food Glorious Food" - from <u>Oliver</u>

Touch - grapes, bananas, loaf of bread, cans of vegetables, etc.

Smell - any of the above or others you may think of

Taste - same as "Smell"

MONDAY'S PLAN:

Show slides/pictures. Talk about the different types of food represented. Use each resident's name frequently. Ask simple questions, for example: "Mr. John Smith, have you ever eaten raw oysters? Mrs. Bessie Jones, did you bake your own bread?" etc.

TUESDAY'S PLAN:

Repeat Monday. End the class with the music. Sing along with it, clap hands. Stretch arms out, up, down, etc. Stretch legs, then kick in time to the beat. Encourage residents to follow your lead. Reward appropriate responses with much praise.

WEDNESDAY'S PLAN:

Repeat Monday's plan. Then add the props. Bring out the fruit, vegetables, loaf of bread, etc. one at a time. Talk about each object. Allow the residents to hold each object in turn. Discuss shape, weight, etc. Discuss the basic food group it may represent. Encourage residents to become involved in the discussion by asking questions like "Mr. John Smith, tell me something about grapes ..." After discussing each object, play the music. Sing along and do the movement exercises as in Tuesday's plan.

THURSDAY'S PLAN:

(For the purpose of this text, it is assumed you have chosen bananas as the food item for smell and taste.) Repeat Wednesday's plan through holding of the food objects, using the banana last. Allow each resident the opportunity to hold the banana, then peel the banana half way down, holding it yourself near each resident's nose asking each to smell deeply. Discuss the banana scent, talk about the heavy smell of banana that fills the air when banana bread is baked. Then slice the banana, giving each resident a slice of banana to taste. Again, discuss the texture in the mouth, the sweet banana taste, etc. Ask each resident to tell a story about the first time each remembers eating a banana. Ask questions about where he/she may have been, who gave them the banana, whether or not he/she likes bananas, etc. Complete the exercise using the music, singing along and/or clapping in beat. Don't forget to do the stretching and kicking portions.

FRIDAY'S PLAN:

Repeat Thursday. Add a sliver of banana cake after tasting the fresh banana. Talk about the banana flavor of the cake and compare the differences between the cake and fresh banana.

EVALUATION OF THE WEEK:

Record each resident's overall response to the week's plan. Answer the following questions about each resident's response:

1. Did he/she track my movements with his/her eyes? ... seem to pay attention?

2. Did he/she seem to repeat the names of the different foods shown? ... recognize the names of the foods? ... seem able to put the names together with the actual food items?

3. Did he/she seem to notice the difference in the different textures of foods handled? ... tasted?

4. Did he/she move in time to the music? ... independent of me? ... with assistance?

5. Did he/she seem to have fun? What portion of this week's program did he/she seem to enjoy most? ... the slides? ... the music? ... the touch of the different food items? ... the smell? ... or, the taste?

6. Did he/she verbalize preferences in foods, i.e., was he/she able to name his/her favorite foods?

WEEK # 10 AND WEEK # 16

THEME: Fruit

OBJECTIVE: Resident will be able to identify and name three different fruits.

MATERIALS TO BE GATHERED:

Vision - slides/pictures of apples, bananas, grapes, oranges, cherries, strawberries, etc.

Hearing - (music) "Banana Boat Song" (Harry Belafonte, circa early '50's)

Touch - at least three of the above mentioned fruits

Smell - fruit jam (strawberry, blackberry, plum, grape, orange marmalade, etc.)

Taste - same as for "Smell"

MONDAY'S PLAN:

Show the slides/pictures. Talk about the different types of fruit represented. Use each resident's name frequently. Use the names of the fruits. Discuss the colors of the fruits, the shapes, how each grows, parts of the country which are famous for growing the fruits, etc. Ask questions about the fruits. Example: "Mr. Jones, have you ever picked an orange in an orange orchard?" "Mrs. Smith, did you ever bake a cherry pie?" etc.

TUESDAY'S PLAN:

Repeat Monday. Add the music at the end of the discussion about the different fruits. Begin moving in time with the music, encourage residents to move with you. Do the arm stretches, and leg stretches as for the preceding week. Clap in time to the music, incorporate the stretches with the hand claps, i.e., clap, stretch; clap, kick; clap, stretch; clap, kick; etc.

WEDNESDAY'S PLAN:

Repeat Monday's plan. Then introduce the different real fruits. Allow each resident to hold the different pieces of fruit. Discuss the texture and shape. Compare the colors of the actual fruit to the colors of the pictures shown. Ask questions about the fruits. Example: "Mr. Jones, this is an apple and this is an orange, - you are holding a lemon. Which fruit is most like the lemon, - the apple or the orange?" "What ingredients are needed to bake a cherry pie?" etc. Then conclude with the music and the movements as per Tuesday's plan.

THURSDAY'S PLAN:

(Have pre-prepared samples of the chosen jams in fluted medicine cups. Also, have coffee stirs ready for the tasting.) Repeat Wednesday's plan through the discussion of the fruits. Bring out the prepared jams and allow each resident an opportunity to smell the jams one at a time. It might be fun to have the residents identify the jams by looking at the color, then smelling the jam. Allow each to taste the jams using the individual coffee stirs for each taste. Ask each resident to tell you something about each of the jams sampled. End with the music and the movement.

FRIDAY'S PLAN:

Repeat Thursday, broadening the questions about the different jams sampled. Allow each resident an opportunity to talk.

EVALUATION OF THE WEEK:

Record each resident's overall response to the week. Answer questions like the following about each participant:

1. Did he/she seem to pay attention to the slides/pictures shown? ... seem to recognize the different fruits?

2. Was he/she able to name the different fruits? ... able to talk about the differences between the fruits?

3. Was he/she anxious to hold the fruits? ... feel the textures and verbalize same?
4. Did each resident seem to participate actively to the best of his/her ability?
5. Did each seem to enjoy the exercises?
6. Does the week bear repeating? ... with different fruits or the same?

*Hint: Adding a drop of lemon juice to the jams will enhance a fresh fruit flavor and scent.

By now, your residents should be responding to this attention. Continue similar programs using weeks planned around:

Vegetables* - Week 11

Meats* - Week 12

Starches* - Week 13

Dairy Products* - Week 14

At the end of each week, evaluate each resident's response to the program. Ask yourself questions like:

1. Did he/she pay attention? ... follow each exercise and track my movement around the area with his/her eyes?
2. Did he/she seem to verbalize the names of the different foods? ... recognize the pictures and match the pictures with the appropriate name of the food?
3. Did he/she move with the music? ... move independently, or did he/she need help moving?
4. Did he/she accomplish the week's goal?
5. Did he/she seem to have fun with the week's program? What part did he/she seem to enjoy most? ... least?
6. Is it time to move on, or should the week be repeated?

* See the listing of materials needed for each week's program which follows.

WEEK #11 AND WEEK #17

THEME: Vegetables

OBJECTIVE: Residents will be able to name and identify three (five) different vegetables.

MATERIALS TO BE GATHERED:

Vision - slides/pictures of carrots, cabbage, spinach, squash, lima beans, etc. At least six different vegetables.

Hearing - (music) recording* of the "Jolly Green Giant" jingle - repeated 4 or 5 times.

Touch - head of cabbage, bunch of carrots, onion, spinach leaf (fresh), squash (assorted types), etc.

Smell - strained Gerber's carrots, strained peas, etc. - sample prepared in fluted medicine cups

Taste - same as for "Smell". Have coffee stirs, individual for each resident times the number of vegetables to be sampled. Example: If plan to sample three vegetables and have ten participants, you will need 30 coffee stirs.

* In recording commercials you may wish to spend quite a bit of time actually recording from your TV or you may wish to solicit the help of a local youth choir from a church or a school and ask them to put together an arrangement that you can tape while they sing; or, you may wish to sing yourself - the talent displayed is not as essential as the message in the music and the beat to which you lead the movement portion of the exercise. You should have at least four minutes of recorded music.

WEEK # 12 AND WEEK # 18

THEME: Meat

OBJECTIVE: Resident will be able to name three different kinds of meat and name the source of the meat, i.e., pork comes from pigs, etc.

MATERIALS TO BE GATHERED:

Vision - pictures/slides of cows, pigs, chickens, lambs, etc. Also pictures of hamburger, steaks, roast and or fried chicken, etc.

Hearing - (music) recording of local hamburger jingles, i.e., for Burger King, MacDonalds's etc.

Touch - toy stuffed animals as listed for vision - minimum of three

Smell -
Taste - } samples of strained meats (particularly if participants are NG tube feeders or if participants are on pureed and/or otherwise mechanically altered diets. If chewing is not a problem, use small bits of whole meats - fried chicken: one whole piece to smell and one additional piece broken into many small tastes.

Remember: One object of this program is to help stimulate the appetite. Work with your dietary department. Explain the objective of each week before beginning and solicit their assistance in preparing the materials needed for "smell" and "taste". Since many residents in need of this sort of program also need encouragement and/or stimulation to eat, your Food Service Supervisor and Dietitian should be informed and involved in the weeks that center around food.

WEEK # 13 AND WEEK # 19

THEME: Starches and Cereals (Grains)

OBJECTIVE: Resident will be able to recognize and name three starches and/or cereals

MATERIALS TO BE GATHERED:

Vision - pictures/slides of potatoes, potato farmers, wheat, corn, oats, different kinds of cereals, breads, rolls, etc.

Hearing - (music) recording of several cereal commercial jingles end to end for at least 4 minutes of music

Touch - ears of corn, shafts of wheat, potatoes, etc.

Smell - corn bread, slice of bread, cooked oatmeal, soda crackers

Taste - same as for "smell". Have samples prepared in advance.

Remember: Some older people have a decreased amount of moisture in their mouths. Be sure to follow the "tastes" with several good swallows of water.

WEEK # 14 AND WEEK # 20

THEME: Dairy Products

OBJECTIVE: Resident will be able to identify and name three dairy products and their source.

MATERIALS TO BE GATHERED:

Vision - pictures/slides of cows, goats, milk, cheeses, milk shakes, ice cream, etc.

Hearing - (music) tape of cows "mooing", goats "nannying" *

Touch - toy cows, goats

Smell - milk, strong cheese, ice cream (flavored)

Taste - ice cream pre-prepared in small medicine cups - several flavors could be fun!

* Tape can be made by yourself making these animal sounds. Follow it with a recording of "Old MacDonald Had a Farm" for the movement and exercise portions.

After going through the weeks entitled "Food," "Fruits," "Vegetables," "Meats," "Starches," "Dairy Products" (weeks 9 - 14) it is appropriate to repeat this six week series to ensure a minimum of at least 50% awareness of residents participating. At that point your residents will be ready to move into some problem solving type activities.

Problem solving activities begin to introduce abstract ideas. The most logical sequence to follow the 12 weeks of basic food types would, of course, be -- meal planning.

LEVEL THREE

WEEK # 21

THEME: Meals, Meal Planning

OBJECTIVE: Residents will be able to plan one meal.

MATERIALS TO BE GATHERED:

Vision - pictures/slides from all four food groups; include a wide variety of pictures

Hearing - (music) "I Wish I Were an Oscar Mayer Weiner", and other similar commercial jingles for food products

Touch -
Smell -
Taste - } variety of raw vegetables, fruits, loaf of bread, meats, protein items, etc. - whatever can be borrowed from your dietary department. Have samples of pureed items available in taste cups (fluted medicine cups) and an equal number of coffee stirs per participant, per taste.

WEEK # 22

THEME: Daytime vs. Nighttime

OBJECTIVE: Residents will be able to identify day from night.

MATERIALS TO BE GATHERED:

Vision - Pictures/slides of daytime and of night time; include panorama type shots

Hearing - (music) "Starry, Starry Night" (Vincent's Song), "Blue Skies Smiling at Me", etc.

Touch - embossed pictures with the sun for day* and with the moon and stars for night*, (discuss the warmth of the sun and the cool of the evening.

Smell - fresh cut grass; warm, damp earth; sunny smells of citrus juices

Taste - pineapple juice, orange juice, etc.

* If embossed pictures are not available make your own using cutouts glued and layered on a background picture.

WEEK # 23

THEME: Numbers

OBJECTIVE: Residents will be able to identify numbers; add simple numbers.

MATERIALS TO BE GATHERED:

Vision - pictures/slides/flash cards* of numbers - variety; pictures of one apple, two bananas, etc.**

Hearing - (music) "One is the Loneliest Number", "One, Two Buckle My Shoe ...", etc.

Touch - plastic or cardboard cut numbers

Smell - samples of the fruits used on the numbered flash cards

* Flash cards can be made on 3 x 5 or 4 x 6 index cards. It is recommended you use unruled cards.

** Like the number flash cards, you can make your own "fruit number" flash cards. Draw and color the fruits in the appropriate colors.

Taste - M & M's - counting the tastes and/or sample tastes of fruits used on the flash cards

WEEK # 24

THEME: Letters, the Alphabet

OBJECTIVE: Residents will be able to identify different letters of the alphabet.

MATERIALS TO BE GATHERED:

Vision - pictures/slides; cardboard letters/plastic letters/flashcards

Hearing - (music) the Alphabet song; "A You're Adorable, B You're so Beautiful".

Touch - cut-outs of letters, plastic letters, etc.

Smell - "A" - apple juice, "B" smashed banana, etc. using 4 or 5 different samples of similar items.

Taste - same as for "Smell"

WEEK # 25

THEME: Names

OBJECTIVE: Residents will be able to identify their own names; the names of one (two) others.

MATERIALS TO BE GATHERED:

Vision - pictures/slides/flashcards with names of people and/or things printed with the picture*

Hearing - (music) "The Name Game"

* Recommend using a few pictures of different types of foods like apple, bananas, etc.

Touch -
Smell -
Taste -   flash cards with letters of alphabet (one per card)**; also letters to spell names of simple foods that will be used for "Smell" and for "Taste". Example: "M" "I" "L" "K", "S" "U" "G" "A" "R", etc

** Use these flashcards as follows: give each resident enough cards to spell his/her first name. Have the resident arrange the cards in the proper order. Example: letters "N" "A" "J" "E" given to resident Jane. Jane is then encouraged and/or helped to arrange the letters to spell her name -"J""A""N""E".

WEEK # 26

THEME: Winter

OBJECTIVE: Residents will be able to name one (two, three) characteristics of winter.

MATERIALS TO BE GATHERED:

Vistion -   pictures/slides of your countryside in winter; pictures/slides of snow, people dressed in coats, etc. Hearing -(music) "Button Up Your Overcoat"

Touch -   soft wool coat

Smell -   the wool coat, hot chocolate, and 2 or 3 other food items associated with winter.

Taste -   the food items used for "Smell".

WEEK # 27

THEME: Summer

OBJECTIVE: Residents will be able to name one (two, three) characteristics of summer.

MATERIALS TO BE GATHERED:

Vision - pictures/slides of your countryside in summer season; pictures/slides of the beach with people in bathing suits, pursuing other leisure activities that occur in summer.

Hearing - "The Long Hot Summer", "In the Summertime", "Summertime and the Living is Easy"

Touch - whole pineapples, bathing suits, water skis, etc.

Smell - pineapple juice, chlorine water of a swimming pool, etc.

Taste - pineapple juice, prune juice,* etc.

* If prune juice is used, discuss how the hot summer sun ripens the fruit.

WEEK # 28

THEME: Spring

OBJECTIVE: Residents will be able to name one (two, three) characteristics of spring.

MATERIALS TO BE GATHERED:

Vision - pictures/slides of your countryside in springtime; pictures of trees budding, plants with new growth, etc.

Hearing - (music) "Red, Red Robin Comes Bob, Bob, Bobbin' Along", "Springtime in the Rockies"

Touch -
Smell - } flowers, plants budding, etc.

Taste - fruits and/or juices of fruits that are representative of pictures of flowering fruit trees shown for the visual portion.

WEEK # 29

THEME: Autumn

OBJECTIVE: Residents will be able to name one (two, three) characteristics of autumn.

MATERIALS TO BE GATHERED:

Vision - pictures/slides of your countryside in autumn; pictures/slides of trees turning colors, etc.

Hearing - (music) "Tenderly"

Touch - leaves that have turned for the fall*

Smell - maple syrup, cane syrup, honey**

Taste - same as for "Smell"

* If this program does not occur during the time of year when you have access to naturally turned leaves, seek silk leaves that represent a fall color scheme.

** Discuss how the plants from which these syrups come are tapped and/or crushed in the fall of the year, or how honey is gathered all summer by the bees and harvested in the fall of the year.

THE "HOLIDAY SERIES"

Tne next eight weeks of program ideas have to do with eight major holidays celebrated in many areas of the country. If the program is continued in the sequence represented in this text, it is strongly recommended that each day the group leader stress the fact that the actual date of the day is not the holiday theme currently under study. Example statements might include, "Today is March 22. It is not Christmas. But, we will discuss Christmas today." Each of these sessions should be similarly closed with a statement such as... "We sang Christmas carols today, but it is not Christmas time. It is, in fact, March 22..."

It is not necessary to use this portion of the program in sequence with the other weeks. You may wish to do these next eight at a time of year that is appropriate for each. You may also wish to add other holidays, particularly those that are familiar to your residents.

WEEK # 30

THEME: New Year's

OBJECTIVE: Residents will be able to discuss New Year's celebrations in which he/she have participated.

MATERIALS TO BE GATHERED:

- Vision - pictures/slides that are representative of this holiday.
- Hearing - (music) "Auld Lang Syne", Spike Jones' "This is my New Year's Resolution".
- Touch - hats, horns, streamers, etc., may be used in celebration at New Year's parties.
- Smell - sparkling grape juice or champagne if permitted in your facility.
- Taste - same as for "Smell"

WEEK # 31

THEME: Valentine's Day

OBJECTIVE: Residents will be able to discuss Valentine's Day

MATERIALS TO BE GATHERED:

- Vision - pictures/slides of couples, people together looking lovingly at each other - as many as can be located.
- Hearing - (music) "Funny Valentine", "Your Cheating Heart", etc.

Touch -	kiss on forehead or cheek; discuss the warm feelings that kissing brings
Smell -	chocolate kisses
Taste -	chocolate kisses

WEEK # 32

THEME: Mardi Gras (for my friends in Mobile, Alabama; Galveston and Austin, Texas; and of course, New Orleans...)

OBJECTIVE: Residents will be able to discuss different types of Mardi Gras celebrations.

MATERIALS TO BE GATHERED:

Vision -	pictures/slides of Mardi Gras in New Orleans, people in costume, the parades, the grand balls, etc.
Hearing -	(music) "Mardi Gras Mambo"
Touch -	Mardi Gras beads and trinkets
Smell -	popcorn, candy apples, hot dogs
Taste -	any of the above that can be digested by the participants.

WEEK # 33

THEME: Easter

OBJECTIVE: Residents will be able to discuss the reasons Easter is celebrated.

MATERIALS TO BE GATHERED:

Vision - pictures of church goers on Easter morning, religious pictures of Easter, children on

	Easter Egg hunts, etc.
Hearing -	(music) "Here Comes Peter Cotton Tail", any of the religious hymns associated with Easter.
Touch -	toy stuffed bunny rabbits, Easter baskets, silk Easter lilies, etc.
Smell -	Easter candy, ham, any food item related to Easter, or flowers related to Easter
Taste -	any of the above food items that can be digested by the participants

WEEK # 34

THEME: 4th of July

OBJECTIVE: Residents will be able to discuss one (two, three) aspects of 4th of July celebrations.

MATERIALS TO BE GATHERED:

Vision -	pictures/slides of the signing of the Constitution; of the American Revolution; 4th of July parades and other celebrations
Hearing -	(music) "Yankee Doodle Dandy"
Touch -	apples, whole watermelon (if in season); straw hat with red, white and blue band; other symbols of the 4th.
Smell -	apple pie or watermelon
Taste -	apple pie or watermelon

WEEK # 35

THEME: Halloween

OBJECTIVE: Residents will be able to discuss past celebrations of Halloween.

MATERIALS TO BE GATHERED:

- Vision - pictures/slides of Halloween, i.e., children trick or treating, illustrations of witches, Icabod Crane, etc.
- Hearing - (music) "Witchcraft"; reading of "Sleepy Hollow"
- Touch - toy, stuffed black cat; witch's hat; pumpkins (if in season), etc.
- Smell - pumpkin pie or pudding; Halloween candy
- Taste - same as "Smell" - keep in mind that only small tastes are enough to satisfy this portion of the program.

WEEK # 36

THEME: Thanksgiving

OBJECTIVE: Residents will be able to discuss the reason Thanksgiving is celebrated in America.

MATERIALS TO BE GATHERED:

- Vision - pictures/slides of the first Thanksgiving; people celebrating Thanksgiving; children's Thanksgiving pageants, etc.
- Hearing - (music) "America, America", "My Country Tis of Thee"

Touch -	Indian corn, feathers, ceramic pilgrims and/or turkeys, yams, etc.
Smell -	popcorn, slice of turkey, yams (baked)
Taste -	any of the above foods within the dietary limitations of participants

WEEK # 37

THEME: Christmas

OBJECTIVE: Residents will share three favorite Christmas memories.

MATERIALS TO BE GATHERED:

Vision -	pictures/slides of the nativity, Christmas trees, people shopping, wrapping gifts, etc.
Hearing -	(music) any Christmas carol or song
Touch -	colorful gifts wrapped for Christmas, Christmas ornaments and/or other seasonal decorations.
Smell -	cranberry juice, apple cider (spiced hot apple juice), etc. (Peppermint is associated with Christmas in many areas of the country.)
Taste -	any of the above items used for "Smell"

"PEOPLE, MEMBERS OF THE FAMILY"

For the next five weeks the general theme will be "People - Members of the Family". This series presents the basic members of the immediate family, i.e., parents, children, mothers, and fathers. You may wish to extend this series by adding the members of an extended family, i.e., grandparents, aunts, uncles, cousins, etc.

WEEK # 38

THEME: People

OBJECTIVE: Residents will identify different (one, two, or three) types of people pictured.

MATERIALS TO BE GATHERED:

- Vision - pictures/slides of people in groups, in couples, alone, different ages working and/or playing together, etc.
- Hearing - (music) "People"
- Touch - dolls that are life-like (not caricatures), figures of life-like people, etc.
- Smell - shoes, clothing, perfumes, etc.
- Taste - "It's a Boy" or "It's a Girl" candy cigars; gingerbread cookies; people shaped cookies

WEEK # 39

THEME: Parents

OBJECTIVE: Residents will be able to discuss one (two, three) helpful hints for young parents.

MATERIALS TO BE GATHERED:

- Vision - couples with children; couples with pregnant woman; mothers with children; Norman Rockwell prints of parent and child
- Hearing - (music) "Is This the Little Girl I Carried" from <u>Fiddler on the Roof</u>; talk about parenthood
- Touch - have residents who are parents participate by holding hands; figurines of parent and child

Smell - cinnamon, Old Spice, smells that remind you of your own parents; discuss what smells remind each resident of their own parents

Taste - chicken soup, milk

WEEK # 40

THEME: Mothers

OBJECTIVE: Residents will discuss their roles as mothers or their own mothers.

MATERIALS TO BE GATHERED:

Vision - pictures/slides of mother's with children, pictures of your residents with their children*

Hearing - (music) The Mother's Day Song, "Ma, He's Making Eyes at Me", "My Momma Said" from <u>Stop the World, I Want to Get Off</u>.

Touch - apron, washboard, etc.**

Smell - cinnamon, apple pie

Taste - same as for "Smell"

* This is a great way to get your families involved in this program.

** Remember: Your residents were mothers and/or had a mother long before the days of women's lib.

WEEK # 41

THEME: Fathers

OBJECTIVE: Residents will discuss their roles as fathers or their own fathers.

MATERIALS TO BE GATHERED:

- Vision - pictures/slides of fathers with children; pictures from the resident's family of the fathers in their family
- Hearing - (music) "Oh, My Papa" (Eddie Fisher, circa 1950's), "Papa I Love You" from <u>Yentil</u>
- Touch - shoes, hat, pipe, folded newspaper
- Smell - cigar (even unlit tobacco has an aroma), coffee, other scents associated with fathers
- Taste - any above food items that may be used for "Smell"

WEEK # 42

THEME: Children

OBJECTIVE: Residents will discuss their own children or children they have known.

MATERIALS TO BE GATHERED:

- Vision - pictures/slides of children of all ages in school, at home, at play, etc.* Pictures of each resident participating when he/she was a child.

* There are some really great Norman Rockwell prints of children in a wide variety of activities.

Hearing - (music) "Is This the Little Girl I Carried" from *Fiddler on the Roof*

Touch - have volunteers bring in a real, live baby**; baby dolls, baby clothes, children's clothing

Smell - baby powder and/or baby oil; crayons; any scent associated with children or childhood; baby foods; etc.

Taste - milk, or any food item that may be introduced in the "Smell" session

** This may not be possible for the three days where "Touch" is used as part of the program, but would be a great follow-up to the week on Friday.

GENERAL THEMES

The last remaining series introduces general themes that cover such basics as trees, flowers, modes of transportation, sports, etc. You may wish to continue to expand this series by developing your own general themes. Other ideas might include different professions such as doctors, lawyers, engineers, farmers, plumbers, etc.; different types of animals such as monkeys, horses, fish, birds, etc.; and a variety of other such concrete themes. Only your imagination limits the number of different weekly themes you develop.

After your residents have participated in this program for a year you should be able to involve some of the participants in the activity program planned for alert/active residents. Others will need to continue in this program indefinitely. At times you may find it to your advantage to repeat all or portions of Level One, particularly if a high number of new residents are introduced to the program at one time.

Perhaps one of the most important components, if not - the most- important component of this program, is your own enthusiasm for it. It just cannot be stressed too much: if you have fun with this, your residents will have fun with it -- and half the battle is won! Because once the residents pay attention enough to enjoy the program time spent with you, they will:

1. build their own attention spans;

2. feel good about their own participation, and

3. begin to feel good about themselves once again.

WEEK # 43

THEME: Trees

OBJECTIVE: Residents will be able to identify one (two, three) trees native to this region.

MATERIALS TO BE GATHERED:

- Vision - pictures/slides of different kinds and types of trees - in all seasons
- Hearing - (music) "Honey" (See the Tree How Big it's Grown), "Tie a Yellow Ribbon", etc., other songs that mention and or name trees.
- Touch - leaves from a variety of different trees
- Smell - pine scent (pine boughs)
- Taste - cookies that are leaf shaped (or candy that is leaf shaped)

WEEK # 44

THEME: Flowers

OBJECTIVE: Residents will be able to identify the names of one (two, three) flowers.

MATERIALS TO BE GATHERED:

- Vision - pictures/slides of a variety of flowers
- Hearing - (music) "Red Roses for a Blue Lady", Theme from <u>The Rose</u>, "Roses are Red My Love, Violets are Blue".
- Touch - fresh flowers - a variety of at least three; if fresh are not available use silk flowers that are sprayed with their scent.

Smell - same as for "Touch"

Taste - candy violets

WEEK # 45

THEME: Boats

OBJECTIVE: Residents will be able to name two (three, four) different types of boats.

MATERIALS TO BE GATHERED:

Vision - pictures/slides of different sizes and types of boats, ships, etc.

Hearing - (music) "Red Sails in the Sunset", "Columbus Sailed the Ocean Blue", Theme from the Love Boat.

Touch - small toy boats (wooden)

Smell - lemon oil on wooden boat

Taste - boat shaped cake; boat shaped candies; cookies that are boat shaped*

* You may wish to purchase a variety of cookie cutter shapes and request a volunteer and/or your dietary department to bake a sugar cookie utilizing the shapes for the weeks where this item is suggested. Remember: You will need enough cookies for Thursday and Friday of each of these weeks, i.e., the number of partici- pants times two (for Thursday and Friday.)

WEEK # 46

THEME: Cars

OBJECTIVE: Residents will be able to name one (two, three) different types of cars.

MATERIALS TO BE GATHERED:

- Vision -   pictures/slides of cars - all types, colors, and sizes
- Hearing -   (music) "Nash Rambler"; tape of automobile commercial jingles
- Touch -   toy cars
- Smell -   motor oil and/or gasoline - on cotton in baby food jar.
- Taste -   candy shaped like cars; cookies shaped like cars

WEEK # 47

THEME: Trains

OBJECTIVE: Residents will be able to identify passenger trains and freight trains and discuss the differences.

MATERIALS TO BE GATHERED:

- Vision -   pictures/slides of different types and kinds of trains
- Hearing -   (music) "Chattanooga Choo Choo"
- Touch -   toy train

Smell - coal. Discuss how trains were once operated by the energy that came from coal burning engines.

Taste - cookies shaped like train cars

WEEK #48

THEME: Airplanes

OBJECTIVE: Residents will be able to identify airplanes, jets, and space vehicles

MATERIALS TO BE GATHERED:

Vision - pictures/slides of airplanes, jets, etc.

Hearing - (music) "Come Fly With Me", "Magnificent Men in Their Flying Machines"

Touch - toy airplane

Smell - gasoline (on cotton in a baby food jar)

Taste - airplane shaped cookies and/or candies

WEEK # 49

THEME: Books, Magazines, Newspapers

OBJECTIVE: Residents will discuss their favorite reading pastimes.

MATERIALS TO BE GATHERED:

Vision - pictures/slides of different types of books, magazines, newspapers or the actual objects.

Hearing - (music) any easily recognized talking book

Touch - books (hard cover and soft cover), magazines, newspaper, etc.

Smell - same as for "Touch"

Taste - book shaped candies and/or cookies

WEEK # 50

THEME: Sports

OBJECTIVE: Residents will be able to identify one (two, three, four) different sports

MATERIALS TO BE GATHERED:

Vision - pictures/slides of different sorts/types of sports

Hearing - (music) Olympic music; "Take Me Out to the Ball Game"; "You've Got to be a Football Hero"; etc.

Touch - baseball, football, bowling ball, golf ball, etc.; a variety of the tools of the different sports illustrated as for "Vision".

Smell - same as for "Touch"

Taste - cookies that are shaped like different sorts of sport balls.

WEEK # 51

THEME: Baseball

OBJECTIVE: Residents will be able to name two (three) different baseball teams and/or famous baseball players.

MATERIALS TO BE GATHERED:

Vision - pictures/slides of different teams; baseball heroes, etc.; baseball cards

Hearing - (music) "Take Me Out to the Ball Game"

Touch - baseball and bat; local team hat and/or uniform

Smell - same as for "Touch"

Taste - cookies shaped like a baseball and/or baseball players

WEEK # 52

THEME: Football

OBJECTIVE: Residents will be able to name two (three, four) football teams and/or famous football players.

MATERIALS TO BE GATHERED:

Vision - pictures/slides of local teams; professional teams; football cards; etc.

Hearing - (music) local high school and/or college cheering squad giving cheers; "You've Got to be a Football Hero".

Touch - football

Smell - leather; football shoe

Taste - football shaped cookies

POSTSCRIPT

After nearly two years into this program many changes have occurred at Hermann Park Manor. Sandra Dorty, the Activity Coordinator who initially called me in for help planning a program for her confused residents, has moved on to bigger and better things. She is back in school now working towards a degree in nursing.

Cloteil Bolden, to whom the responsibility for carrying out this program fell, is now the chief Activity Coordinator. But this is still her "baby". Her new assistant is handling the routine activities for the more alert, active residents. Cloteil has a special spot in her heart for the many residents who participate in the Sensory Stim classes. And, she has a special talent for reaching the "hard to reach" residents.

The Sensory Stimulation program at Hermann Park Manor has expanded far beyond the ideas presented in this text. What once began with bi-weekly planning sessions meticulously brainstorming ideas and program goals two weeks at a time, has now become a way of life for Cloteil and her special residents.

Mrs. A. S., sadly, passed away a few months ago. But her last year and a half of life had a quality of joy many nursing home residents might envy.

I saw Mr. H. S. this past week on an outing with a number of other residents from Hermann Park Manor. He was talking and enjoying himself, visiting with contestants in the 1987 Greater Ms. Years Pageant* at a local country club. Watching Mr. H. S. at this event put a lump in my throat. It was rewarding to see this man, who two years ago couldn't even sit still long enough to eat a meal, participate in an afternoon outing with more than two hundred other nursing home residents and members of the public.

I have helped to implement this program in a number of other nursing homes since first working with Sandra and Cloteil back in mid 1985. And, have seen several other such "miracles" as Mrs. A. S. and Mr. H. S. It is difficult to assess where the "miracles" may occur -- is it the program? the constant consistent attention? or, the enthusiasm of the different program leaders -- their idea that this program works, therefore it does? Whatever the cause, it does not really matter. What does matter is the quality of life improvement this program and other similar programs may bring to your confused residents.

Use this information and the program ideas to your advantage. Take these progression activity ideas and make them yours -- watch the quality of life for your "Special" residents improve. Use this text as a springboard for your own unique program and let me hear about your "miracles".

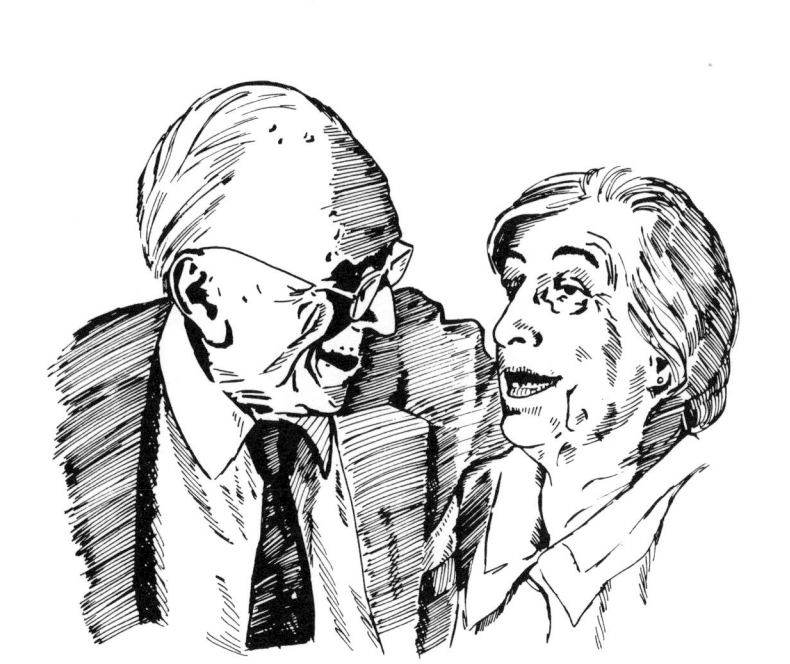

Pamela Powder

* Greater Ms. Years Pageant is a yearly event sponsored by the Greater Houston Chapter of the Texas Health Care Association, a beauty pageant for nursing home residents -- the octogenarian Miss America.

APPENDIX

Sample forms to aid in individual program planning.

(Sample Weekly Planning Page)

WEEK

THEME:

OBJECTIVE:

MATERIALS TO BE GATHERED:

    Vision -

    Hearing - (music)

    Touch -

    Smell

    Taste

MONDAY'S PLAN:

TUESDAY'S PLAN:

WEDNESAY'S PLAN:

THURSDAY'S PLAN:

FRIDAY'S PLAN:

EVALUATION OF WEEK:

(Sample Resident Participation Record Form)

SENSORY STIMULATION
RESIDENT'S PARTICIPATION RECORD

Week of _____ Theme of Week _____

R - responded   A - active

O - no participation   P - passive

Residents' Names	M	T	W	Th	F	Comments